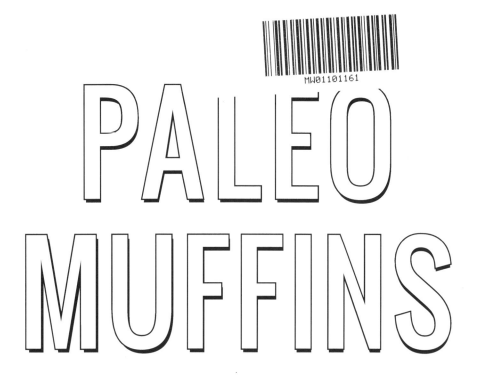

PALEO MUFFINS

Gluten-Free Paleo Muffin Recipes for a Paleo Diet

||||||||||||||||||||||||||||||||||||||||||||||||

By John Chatham

For general information on our other products and services or to obtain technical support, please contact our Customer Care Department within the U.S. at (866) 744-2665, or outside the U.S. at (510) 253-0500.

Rockridge University Press publishes its books in a variety of electronic and print formats. Some content that appears in print may not be available in electronic books, and vice versa.

ISBN: Print 978-1-62315-096-9 | eBook 978-1-62315-097-6

CONTENTS

Introduction   1

Section One: Gluten-Free Paleo Muffins   3

Chapter 1: Breakfast Muffins

Paleo Blueberry Muffins   4

Paleo Morning Muffins   6

Paleo "Bran" Muffins   8

Cinnamon-Raisin Muffins with Walnut Streusel   9

"Oatmeal" Muffins   11

Apple Cranberry Breakfast Muffins   12

Bacon and Roasted Pepper Muffins   13

French Toast Muffins   14

Paleo Morning Glory Muffins   16

Pecan Date Muffins   17

Chai Spiced Muffins   18

Chapter 2: Fruit and Vegetable Muffins

Apple Cinnamon Muffins   19

Paleo Pumpkin Muffins   21

Paleo Carrot Muffins 22

Paleo Banana-Nut Muffins 24

Paleo Zucchini Muffins 25

Vanilla-Cinnamon Applesauce Muffins 26

Honey Peach Muffins 27

Pineapple Muffins 28

Raspberry Muffins 29

Spiced Sweet Potato Muffins 30

Mango Muffins 31

Cranberry Orange Muffins 32

Cherry Almond Muffins 33

Chapter 3: Dessert Muffins

Paleo Almond Muffins 34

Lemon Poppy Seed Muffins 36

Paleo Honey Muffins 37

Simple Chocolate Muffins 38

Maple Pecan Muffins 39

Chocolate Almond Butter Muffins 40

Vanilla Almond Muffins 42

Chocolate Coconut Muffins 43

Blueberry Chocolate Chip Mini Muffins 44

Double-Chocolate Cherry Muffins 46

Double-Chocolate Peppermint Muffins 48

Key Lime Coconut Muffins   49

Browned-Butter Honey Muffins   50

Chocolate Chip Banana Muffins   51

Section Two: The Basics of the Paleo Diet   **52**

Chapter 4: What Is the Paleo Diet?   **53**

Chapter 5: The Benefits of Paleo   **57**

Chapter 6: The Trouble with Gluten   **61**

Chapter 7: Paleo Food Guide   **66**

Conclusion   **71**

Resources   **73**

INTRODUCTION

Piping hot and deliciously decadent, muffins are without a doubt one of the tastiest baked confections on the planet. Depending on what you bake into them, muffins are great for breakfast, with tea, as a midmorning snack, or as a scrumptious dessert. Sister to the cupcake, the muffin often appeals to those who prefer something with just a bit of sweetness, but without the decadence of icing and filling. Since they're easy to hold and are made in single-serving portions, they're also popular with those constantly on the go.

Unfortunately the muffin doesn't generally favor a healthful, low-calorie diet, and since it typically contains white sugar, processed and gluten-rich flour, and additives like chocolate chips, most diets, including the Paleo diet, typically forbid them entirely. That is, until now.

You see, the reason your standard muffin makes the no-no list for healthful eaters is precisely because it contains the trifecta of bad foods: white sugar, processed flour, and bad fats. All of these contribute to such diseases and disorders as heart disease, diabetes, celiac disease, and obesity. It's no coincidence that these conditions—known as "diseases of excess"—are almost completely exclusive to individuals following the Western diet. But what if you start tweaking the recipes so that good ingredients replace the bad?

That's exactly what was done to the recipes in the following pages. Many people simply aren't willing to give up the scrumptiousness of muffins in the name of good health, so this book does the only other feasible thing: it provides ways to make muffins that are actually healthful additions to a Paleo diet. Some of our favorite gluten-free muffins: Paleo Blueberry Muffins, Paleo Banana-Nut Muffins, and of course, the delicious, nutritious Paleo Pumpkin Muffin.

In the pages to come, you'll learn how to make Paleo breakfast muffins as well as muffins that are great for snacking or desserts. Included are a wide variety of recipes so that no matter what your preferences and favorite flavors are, you'll find something you adore. Without further ado, let's make some muffins!

SECTION ONE
Gluten-Free Paleo Muffins

- **Chapter 1:** Breakfast Muffins

- **Chapter 2:** Fruit and Vegetable Muffins

- **Chapter 3:** Dessert Muffins

BREAKFAST MUFFINS

Paleo Blueberry Muffins

Think you have to give up your morning blueberry muffin just because you've gone Paleo? Think again. These moist muffins bursting with tender and juicy blueberries will satisfy your craving for a coffee shop muffin without the guilt that usually accompanies it. Freeze them for a quick breakfast or sweet treat anytime you want.

- 2 1/2 cups blanched almond flour
- 1 tablespoon coconut flour
- 1 teaspoon baking soda
- 1 teaspoon sea salt
- 1 teaspoon cinnamon
- 1 stick unsalted, grass-fed butter, softened
- 1 cup pure maple syrup
- 2 large eggs
- 2 cups unsweetened applesauce, preferably homemade
- 1/4 cup unsweetened almond milk
- 1 tablespoon pure vanilla extract
- 1 cup fresh or frozen blueberries

Preheat oven to 350 degrees F.

Combine the almond flour, coconut flour, baking soda, salt, and cinnamon in a large bowl. Stir and set aside.

In a mixing bowl, beat the butter with the maple syrup, and add the eggs, beating separately with each egg.

On low speed, add the applesauce, followed by the almond milk and vanilla.

Add the flour mixture, and beat on low until just combined. Carefully fold in the blueberries. Stir gently until well combined.

Line a muffin tin with liners, and fill each cup 2/3 full of batter. Bake for 12–14 minutes, until tops are golden brown. Once cooled, loosen the muffins with a knife and serve.

Store any leftovers in an airtight container for up to 3 days.

Makes 1 dozen muffins.

Paleo Morning Muffins

Looking for something quick and healthful you can grab as you head out the door? These morning muffins will do the trick. Filled with healthful ingredients like dried fruit and nuts, they are a much better choice than the carb-heavy muffins you may get at the donut shop on the way to work. They also freeze extremely well, so just heat them up and go.

- 1/2 cup unsweetened applesauce, preferably homemade
- 2 tablespoons coconut oil, melted
- 1 tablespoon fresh lemon juice
- 1/2 cup unsweetened almond milk
- 1 large egg
- 1 teaspoon pure vanilla extract
- 1 cup blanched almond flour
- 1/4 cup coconut flour
- 1 tablespoon cinnamon
- 1 teaspoon baking soda
- 1/2 teaspoon sea salt
- 1/2 cup unsweetened coconut flakes
- 4 dried apricots, chopped
- 2 tablespoons raisins
- 2 tablespoons walnuts, chopped

Preheat oven to 350 degrees F.

Put the applesauce, coconut oil, lemon juice, almond milk, egg, and vanilla in a bowl, and stir well to combine.

In a separate bowl, whisk together the almond flour, coconut flour, cinnamon, baking soda, and salt. Pour the liquid into the dry mixture, and stir until just combined.

Fold in the coconut flakes, apricots, raisins, and walnuts.

Line a muffin tin with liners, and fill each cup 2/3 full of batter. Bake for 12–14 minutes, until tops are golden brown. Once cooled, loosen the muffins with a knife and serve.

Store any leftovers in an airtight container for up to 3 days.

Makes 1 dozen muffins.

Paleo "Bran" Muffins

While these don't actually contain any bran (bran, also known as "wheat" bran, is the outer bran of the wheat stalk, and not gluten-free or Paleo friendly), flaxseed and molasses give them a similar dark color, texture, and flavor of your favorite coffeehouse bran muffin. This means these include no wheat or refined carbs. Instead, you're getting something delicious, good for you, and as filling as traditional bran muffins but without the wheat belly that comes with it. Try these plain or with Paleo-approved jam for an easy and healthful breakfast.

- 1/2 cup blanched almond flour
- 1/2 cup ground flaxseeds
- 2 tablespoons coconut flour
- 1 teaspoon baking soda
- 1/2 teaspoon sea salt
- 1 tablespoon natural almond butter
- 3 large eggs
- 2 tablespoons molasses
- 1 small ripe banana, mashed
- 1/2 cup unsweetened almond milk

Preheat oven to 350 degrees F.

In a large bowl, combine the almond flour, flax, coconut flour, baking soda, and salt. Set aside.

In a separate bowl, beat together the almond butter, eggs, molasses, mashed banana, and almond milk. Pour the wet ingredients into the flour mixture, and stir until well combined.

Line a muffin tin with liners, and fill each cup 2/3 full of batter. Bake for 12–14 minutes, until tops are golden brown. Once cooled, loosen the muffins with a knife and serve.

Store any leftovers in an airtight container for up to 3 days.

Makes 1 dozen muffins.

Cinnamon-Raisin Muffins with Walnut Streusel

Miss your favorite morning cinnamon roll, or craving a slice of cinnamon-raisin bread? If so, this recipe is sure to become a favorite. These simple-to-prepare muffins are laced with cinnamon and topped with a buttery, walnut topping that will immediately remind you of your favorite bakery treat. These are fabulous for a Paleo-style brunch, and will instantly have your guests wondering how you pulled off such a decadent indulgence that's Paleo friendly. While you can serve them at room temperature, they are best served warm from the oven.

For the muffins:
- 2 cups blanched almond flour
- 1/2 teaspoon sea salt
- 2 teaspoons baking soda
- 4 large eggs
- 1/2 cup unsalted, grass-fed butter, melted and cooled
- 1/4 cup pure honey
- 1/2 cup unsweetened almond milk

For the streusel topping:
- 1/4 cup chopped walnuts
- 2 tablespoons coconut flour
- 2 tablespoons coconut sugar
- 2 tablespoons unsalted, grass-fed butter, cold and cubed

Make the muffins:
Preheat oven to 350 degrees F.

In a large bowl, combine the almond flour, salt, and baking soda. Set aside.

In a mixing bowl, beat the eggs with the melted butter, honey, and almond milk until light and smooth. Pour into the flour mixture, and stir until well combined.

Make the streusel topping:

Add the chopped walnuts, coconut flour, coconut sugar, and cold butter in a small bowl, and crumble the butter into the flour and sugar with your hands until you have a crumbly mixture.

Line a muffin tin with liners, and fill each cup 2/3 full of batter. Top with the streusel topping. Bake for 12–14 minutes, until tops are golden brown. Once slightly cooled, loosen the muffins with a knife and serve warm.

Store any leftovers in an airtight container for up to 3 days. You can freeze these for weeks in a freezer bag for serving anytime.

Makes 1 dozen muffins.

"Oatmeal" Muffins

You've probably heard before that a hot bowl of oatmeal is one of the best ways to start your day; however, if you've gone Paleo, this is no longer an option. These muffins can fulfill your craving for oats even though they don't actually contain any. Finely shredded coconut mimics the texture of oats, while some cinnamon and maple syrup can make you feel like you're enjoying a winter bowl of oatmeal. Although these muffins are acceptable at room temperature, they're best served warm.

- 2 cups blanched almond flour
- 1/2 cup unsweetened coconut, shredded
- 1/2 teaspoon sea salt
- 1 teaspoon cinnamon
- 2 teaspoons baking soda
- 3 large eggs
- 1/2 cup coconut oil, melted
- 1/4 cup pure maple syrup
- 1/2 cup unsweetened almond milk

Preheat oven to 350 degrees F.

In a large bowl, combine the almond flour, coconut, salt, cinnamon, and baking soda. Set aside.

In a mixing bowl, beat the eggs with the coconut oil, maple syrup, and almond milk until light and smooth. Pour into the flour mixture, and stir until well combined.

Line a muffin tin with liners, and fill each cup 2/3 full of batter. Bake for 12–14 minutes, until tops are a deep golden brown. Once cooled, loosen the muffins with a knife and serve.

Store any leftovers in an airtight container for up to 3 days. You can freeze these for weeks in a freezer bag for serving anytime.

Makes 1 dozen muffins.

Apple Cranberry Breakfast Muffins

Looking for something sweet and tart to start your morning? Look no further than these delightful breakfast muffins made with fresh cranberries and apples. Bursting with fresh fruit flavor, these are an easy way to start your day off right. Combining the fresh, chopped cranberries with a bit of coconut sugar prevents them from making your muffins too sour, so be sure to include that step.

- 1/2 cup fresh cranberries
- 2 tablespoons coconut sugar
- 2 tablespoons pure maple syrup
- 1 large egg
- 2 teaspoons pure vanilla extract
- 1 cup unsweetened almond milk
- 1 cup blanched almond flour
- 1/4 teaspoon sea salt
- 1/4 teaspoon baking soda
- 1 apple, peeled, cored, and chopped

Preheat oven to 350 degrees F.

Put the cranberries in a food processor with the coconut sugar. Pulse until the cranberries are chopped and mixed well with the sugar, being careful not to puree them.

In a medium bowl, add the maple syrup, egg, vanilla, and almond milk, and beat to combine.

In a separate bowl, combine the almond flour, salt, and baking soda. Stir well. Add the liquid and stir until well combined. Fold in the chopped cranberries and apples.

Line a muffin tin with liners, and fill each cup 2/3 full of batter. Bake for 12–14 minutes, until tops are golden brown. Serve warm or at room temperature.

Store any leftovers in an airtight container for up to 3 days.

Makes 1 dozen muffins.

Bacon and Roasted Pepper Muffins

These savory breakfast muffins are full of flavor from the crisp, cooked bacon and roasted peppers. With a texture that is light and airy, they are incredibly satisfying yet still manage to stick to the principles of the Paleo diet. They're great when you want something that's simple to grab and go but isn't necessarily sweet. Freeze any remaining for an easy, flavorful breakfast any day of the week.

- 1 cup blanched almond flour
- 1/2 teaspoon sea salt
- 2 teaspoons baking soda
- 6 large eggs
- 1/2 cup unsalted, grass-fed butter, melted and cooled
- 1/2 cup water
- 4–5 slices nitrate-free bacon, cooked until crisp, and crumbled
- 1 roasted red pepper, finely chopped

Preheat oven to 325 degrees F.

In a large bowl, combine the almond flour, salt, and baking soda. Set aside.

Beat the eggs with the melted butter and water. Add in the bacon and roasted peppers. Pour this mixture into the flour mix, and stir until combined.

Line a muffin tin with liners, and fill each cup 2/3 full of batter. Bake for 12–14 minutes, until tops are golden brown. Once cooled, loosen the muffins with a knife and serve.

Store any leftovers in an airtight container for up to 3 days. You can freeze these for weeks in a freezer bag for serving anytime.

Makes 1 dozen muffins.

French Toast Muffins

These amazing French toast muffins require sourcing some Paleo-friendly bread (or making your own), but the result is well worth the effort. If you have a Paleo bread recipe that you like, save a few slices next time you make it in order to try these muffins—you won't be disappointed. These are best served immediately after removing from the oven.

For the topping:

- 1 egg
- 3 tablespoons unsweetened almond milk
- 1 teaspoon pure vanilla
- 1/2 teaspoon cinnamon
- 4 slices Paleo-friendly white bread, cut into small cubes

For the muffins:

- 2 cups blanched almond flour
- 1/2 teaspoon sea salt
- 2 teaspoons baking soda
- 4 large eggs
- 1/2 cup unsalted, grass-fed butter, melted and cooled
- 1/4 cup pure honey
- 1/2 cup unsweetened almond milk
- Pure maple syrup, for brushing the tops

Make the topping:

Beat the egg with the almond milk, vanilla, and cinnamon, and pour over the bread cubes. Set aside.

Make the muffins:

Preheat oven to 350 degrees F.

In a large bowl, combine the almond flour, salt, and baking soda. Set aside.

In a mixing bowl, beat the eggs with the butter, honey, and almond milk until light and smooth. Pour into the flour mixture, and stir until well combined.

Line a muffin tin with liners, and fill each cup 2/3 full of batter. Divide the French toast cubes evenly between the muffins.

Bake for 12–14 minutes, until tops are golden brown and bread cubes are browned around the edges. Brush the tops with maple syrup and serve warm.

Makes 1 dozen muffins.

Paleo Morning Glory Muffins

These dense and delicious muffins are chock-full of goodness, making them perfect for a busy day or a midday snack when you need a burst of energy. Loaded with ingredients like carrots, raisins, and an apple, this is not a cake-like muffin but sweet and full of texture and flavor.

- 2 tablespoons coconut oil, melted
- 1/2 cup unsweetened almond milk
- 1 large egg
- 1 teaspoon pure vanilla extract
- 1 cup almond flour
- 1/4 cup ground flaxseed
- 1/4 cup unsweetened coconut, shredded
- 1 tablespoon cinnamon
- 1/4 teaspoon ground nutmeg
- 1 teaspoon baking soda
- 1 cup carrots, grated
- 1 apple, peeled, cored, and chopped
- 1/4 cup raisins
- 1/2 cup walnuts, chopped

Preheat oven to 350 degrees F.

Put the coconut oil, almond milk, egg, and vanilla in a bowl, and stir well to combine.

In a separate bowl, whisk together the almond flour, flaxseed, coconut, cinnamon, nutmeg, and baking soda. Pour the liquid mixture into the dry mixture, and stir until just combined.

Fold in the carrots, apple, raisins, and walnuts.

Line a muffin tin with liners, and fill each cup 2/3 full of batter. Bake for 12–14 minutes, until tops are dark brown. Once cooled, loosen the muffins with a knife and serve.

Store any leftovers in an airtight container for up to 3 days.

Makes 1 dozen muffins.

Pecan Date Muffins

These muffins are sweetened with dates alone, giving you a nice dose of natural sugar in the morning before you embark on your day. Crunchy pecans throughout add additional flavor to these tasty muffins. You can freeze any leftovers, which make a quick breakfast a breeze when you don't have time to cook or even sit down for a meal. Grab one to go, and it will be thawed out by the time you arrive at the office!

- 2 cups blanched almond flour
- 2 teaspoons baking soda
- 1/2 teaspoon sea salt
- 4 large eggs
- 1/2 cup unsalted, grass-fed butter, melted and cooled
- 1/2 cup unsweetened almond milk
- 1/4 cup dates, pitted and chopped
- 1/2 cup pecans, chopped

Preheat oven to 350 degrees F.

In a large bowl, combine the almond flour, baking soda, and salt. Set aside.

In a mixing bowl, beat the eggs with the butter and almond milk until light and smooth. Pour into the flour mixture, and stir until well combined. Fold in the chopped dates and pecans.

Line a muffin tin with liners, and fill each cup 2/3 full of batter. Bake for 12–14 minutes, until tops are golden brown. Once cooled, loosen the muffins with a knife and serve.

Store any leftovers in an airtight container for up to 3 days. You can freeze these for weeks in a freezer bag for serving anytime.

Makes 1 dozen muffins.

Chai Spiced Muffins

Fragrant with a hint of Indian spices, these delicious Paleo-friendly muffins make an excellent substitute for your usual chai latte. These simple, elegant muffins are perfect for a quick breakfast or sweet snack. These are best served warm with a pat of unsalted, grass-fed butter.

- 2 cups blanched almond flour
- 2 teaspoons baking soda
- 1 teaspoon cinnamon
- 1/2 teaspoon ground ginger
- 1/2 teaspoon ground cardamom
- 1/4 teaspoon freshly ground black pepper
- 1/2 teaspoon sea salt
- 4 large eggs
- 1/2 cup coconut oil, melted
- 1/4 cup pure honey
- 1/2 cup unsweetened almond milk

Preheat oven to 350 degrees F.

In a large bowl, combine the almond flour, baking soda, spices, pepper, and salt. Set aside.

In a mixing bowl, beat the eggs with the coconut oil, honey, and almond milk until light and smooth. Pour into the flour mixture, and stir until well combined.

Line a muffin tin with liners, and fill each cup 2/3 full of batter. Bake for 12–14 minutes, until tops are golden brown. Once cooled, loosen the muffins with a knife and serve.

Store any leftovers in an airtight container for up to 3 days. You can freeze these for weeks in a freezer bag for serving anytime.

Makes 1 dozen muffins.

2

FRUIT AND VEGETABLE MUFFINS

Apple Cinnamon Muffins

There is nothing better than the smell of apples and cinnamon baking in the oven, and these delightfully flavorful muffins will prove that. Eat these warm from the pan with a pat of unsalted, grass-fed butter for a real treat. You can use any type of apple you like here; for sweeter muffins, use a Red Delicious or other sweet variety.

- 2 tablespoons pure maple syrup
- 1 large egg
- 2 teaspoons pure vanilla extract
- 1 cup unsweetened almond milk
- 1 cup blanched almond flour
- 1 teaspoon cinnamon
- 1/4 teaspoon sea salt
- 1/4 teaspoon baking soda
- 1 apple, peeled, cored, and chopped

Preheat oven to 350 degrees F.

In a medium bowl, combine the maple syrup, egg, vanilla, and almond milk, and beat to combine.

In a separate bowl, stir together the almond flour, cinnamon, salt, and baking soda. Add the liquid mixture and stir until well combined. Fold in the chopped apples.

Line a muffin tin with liners, and fill each cup 2/3 full of batter. Bake for 12–14 minutes, until tops are golden brown. Serve warm or at room temperature.

Store any leftovers in an airtight container for up to 3 days.

Makes 1 dozen muffins.

Paleo Pumpkin Muffins

Pureed pumpkin makes these muffins moist and tender, while its fragrant spices make them full of spicy flavor. These are excellent served with unsalted, grass-fed butter, but you'll definitely enjoy them plain as well. Make these in the fall when the aroma will remind you of crisp, chilly days and the upcoming holiday season. They freeze particularly well, so make an extra batch, and have a taste of autumn all year round.

- 1 cup blanched almond flour
- 1/2 cup pecans or walnuts, finely ground
- 1 teaspoon baking soda
- 1 teaspoon cinnamon
- 1/4 teaspoon ground nutmeg
- 1/4 teaspoon ground ginger
- 1/2 teaspoon sea salt
- 1 large egg
- 1 cup pumpkin puree
- 1/2 cup unsweetened almond milk
- 3 tablespoons pure maple syrup

Preheat oven to 350 degrees F.

In a large mixing bowl, stir together the almond flour, ground nuts, baking soda, spices, and salt.

In a small bowl, beat the egg, pumpkin, almond milk, and maple syrup until well combined. Add the wet ingredients to the flour mixture and mix well.

Line a muffin tin with liners, and fill each cup 2/3 full of batter. Bake for 12–14 minutes, until tops are golden brown. Once cooled, loosen the muffins with a knife and serve.

Store any leftovers in an airtight container or loosely wrapped in plastic for up to 3 days.

Makes 1 dozen muffins.

Paleo Carrot Muffins

Moist and tender, these easy-to-prepare carrot muffins will satisfy your cravings for a slice of carrot cake, and you won't be eating all the refined sugar and carbs. You can eat these for breakfast and feel good about it, or simply enjoy them as a sweet treat after a meal. These sweet and spicy muffins are also an excellent addition to a Paleo brunch or other gathering where you'd like a healthful yet indulgent option. You won't miss traditional carrot cake—and the highly sugared frosting that usually adorns it—once you taste these muffins.

- 1/2 cup unsweetened applesauce, preferably homemade
- 2 tablespoons coconut oil, melted
- 1/2 cup unsweetened almond milk
- 1 large egg
- 1 teaspoon pure vanilla extract
- 1 cup blanched almond flour
- 1/4 cup coconut flour
- 1 tablespoon cinnamon
- 1/4 teaspoon ground nutmeg
- 1 teaspoon baking soda
- 1 cup carrots, grated
- 1/2 cup walnuts, chopped
- 1/4 cup raisins

Preheat oven to 350 degrees F.

Put the applesauce, coconut oil, almond milk, egg, and vanilla in a bowl, and stir well to combine.

In a separate bowl, whisk together the almond flour, coconut flour, cinnamon, nutmeg, and baking soda. Pour the liquid ingredients into the dry mixture, and stir until just combined.

Fold in the carrots, walnuts, and raisins.

Line a muffin tin with liners, and fill each cup 2/3 full of batter. Bake for 12–14 minutes, until tops are golden brown. Once cooled, loosen the muffins with a knife and serve.

Store any leftovers in an airtight container for up to 3 days.

Makes 1 dozen muffins.

Paleo Banana-Nut Muffins

There's not much better than a sweet, spicy, banana-laced muffin filled with crunchy walnuts. Unfortunately, most banana-nut muffins are filled with sugar, processed vegetable oils, and refined carbs. Not so with these beauties. They are just as tender and delicious as your favorite coffee shop muffin, but they are actually good for you. You can add some high-quality chocolate chips to these for an extra indulgence, but taste them first—you may find they don't need it. Freeze any leftovers in a plastic bag; they'll keep for weeks as a sweet treat whenever you like.

- 1 cup blanched almond flour
- 1/2 cup coconut flour
- 1 teaspoon baking soda
- 1 teaspoon cinnamon
- 1/2 teaspoon sea salt
- 1 large egg
- 1 cup ripened bananas, mashed
- 1/2 cup unsweetened almond milk
- 3 tablespoons pure maple syrup

Preheat oven to 350 degrees F.

In a large mixing bowl, combine the almond flour, coconut flour, baking soda, cinnamon, and salt. Stir to combine.

In a small bowl, combine the egg, bananas, almond milk, and maple syrup. Beat until well combined. Add the wet ingredients to the flour mixture, and mix well.

Line a muffin tin with liners, and fill each cup 2/3 full of batter. Bake for 12–14 minutes, until tops are golden brown. Once cooled, loosen the muffins with a knife and serve.

Store any leftovers in an airtight container or loosely wrapped in plastic for up to 3 days.

Makes 1 dozen muffins.

Paleo Zucchini Muffins

Have a garden full of zucchini and don't know what to do with them? Normally you'd make zucchini muffins, but since you've gone Paleo, that's out, right? Don't rule it out just yet. With these easy-to-prepare muffins that are moist and full of flavor, there's no need to discard your crop. These are just as delicious as your favorite traditional recipe, but they fit within the Paleo plan. Still convinced it's not possible? Whip up a batch of these and see for yourself.

- 1/2 cup unsweetened applesauce, preferably homemade
- 2 tablespoons coconut oil, melted
- 1/2 cup unsweetened almond milk
- 2 large eggs
- 1 teaspoon pure vanilla extract
- 1 cup blanched almond flour
- 1/4 cup coconut flour
- 1 tablespoon cinnamon
- 1/4 teaspoon ground nutmeg
- 1 teaspoon baking soda
- 1 cup zucchini, grated
- 1/2 cup walnuts, chopped (optional)

Preheat oven to 350 degrees F.

Put the applesauce, coconut oil, almond milk, eggs, and vanilla in a bowl, and stir well to combine.

In a separate bowl, whisk together the almond flour, coconut flour, cinnamon, nutmeg, and baking soda. Pour the liquid ingredients into the dry mixture, and stir until just combined.

Fold in the shredded zucchini, then the walnuts if using.

Line a muffin tin with liners, and fill each cup 2/3 full of batter. Bake for 12–14 minutes, until tops are golden brown. Once cooled, loosen the muffins with a knife and serve.

Store any leftovers in an airtight container for up to 3 days.

Makes 1 dozen muffins.

Vanilla-Cinnamon Applesauce Muffins

Lightly fragrant, these vanilla-scented muffins have a hint of apple flavor, thanks to the applesauce used to bake them. Applesauce not only adds flavor but is great for adding moisture and replacing fat. Do yourself a favor: if you can make some homemade applesauce, do it. The store-bought product is adequate if it's sugar free, but as with anything, there's always a difference when you make it yourself. Try these with some jam or softened unsalted, grass-fed butter, or just enjoy them plain. Either way, these are simply delightful!

- 2 cups blanched almond flour
- 1 tablespoon cinnamon
- 1 teaspoon baking soda
- 2 large eggs
- 1/2 cup cold water
- 1 teaspoon pure vanilla extract
- 1/4 cup pure maple syrup
- 1/2 cup unsweetened applesauce, preferably homemade

Preheat oven to 350 degrees F.

Mix together the almond flour, cinnamon, and baking soda in a bowl, and sift to combine well.

In a large bowl, beat the eggs until they are frothy. Add the water, vanilla, and maple syrup, and beat until well combined. Stir in the applesauce and mix well.

Carefully pour the flour mixture into the wet ingredients, and stir until just combined.

Line a mini muffin tin with liners, or grease lightly with coconut oil, and fill each cup 2/3 full of batter. Bake for 12–14 minutes until golden brown and fragrant with the scent of cinnamon and vanilla. Allow to cool completely before removing from the pan.

Store any remaining muffins in an airtight container for up to 3 days.

Makes 1 dozen muffins.

Honey Peach Muffins

Fragrant peaches turn these muffins into tender delights sure to satisfy any sweet tooth. For the best possible flavor, make these when peaches are in season, and wait until yours are especially ripe—the softer and riper your peaches, the sweeter and more flavorful your muffins will be. Serve these for a Sunday brunch treat, and every guest will be asking for the recipe. These are marvelous with a Paleo-approved raspberry or strawberry jam, but they are equally delicious plain or with just a pat of unsalted, grass-fed butter. Freeze leftovers for an anytime treat the whole family will love.

- 2 cups blanched almond flour
- 1 teaspoon baking soda
- 1/2 teaspoon sea salt
- 2 large eggs
- 1/2 cup cold water
- 1 teaspoon pure vanilla extract
- 1/4 cup pure honey
- 2 medium ripe peaches, pitted, peeled, and finely chopped

Preheat oven to 350 degrees F.

Mix together the almond flour, baking soda, and salt in a bowl, and sift to combine well.

In a large bowl, beat the eggs until they are frothy. Add the water, vanilla, and honey, and beat until well combined.

Carefully pour the flour mixture into the wet ingredients, and stir until just combined. Fold in the peaches, and stir until just mixed.

Line a muffin tin with liners, and fill each cup 2/3 full of batter. Bake for 2–4 minutes until golden brown. Allow to cool before removing from pan.

Store any leftovers in an airtight container for up to 3 days.

Makes 1 dozen muffins.

Pineapple Muffins

With fresh pineapple, shredded coconut, and mashed bananas, these muffins are a tropical delight perfect for an afternoon tea or Sunday brunch. They are excellent served plain, as the pineapple and bananas provide unparalleled moistness with a hint of sweetness. Either fresh or canned pineapple work equally well; if you choose canned, make sure it's packed in water instead of syrup to avoid the added refined sugar typically found in canned fruits. Freeze any remaining muffins in freezer bags for a tropical treat any day of the week.

- 2 cups blanched almond flour
- 2 teaspoons baking soda
- 1 teaspoon sea salt
- 1/4 cup unsweetened coconut, shredded
- 2 large eggs
- 1/2 cup coconut oil
- 1/4 cup pure honey
- 1 cup coconut milk
- 1 small ripe banana, mashed
- 1/2 cup crushed pineapple

Preheat oven to 350 degrees F.

Combine the almond flour, baking soda, salt, and shredded coconut in a large bowl.

In a separate bowl, beat the eggs with the coconut oil, honey, and coconut milk. Stir in the banana.

Add the liquid ingredients to the dry mixture, and stir until well combined. Fold in the pineapple and stir until just combined.

Line a muffin tin with liners, and fill each cup 2/3 full of batter. Bake for 12–14 minutes, until tops are golden brown. Once cooled, loosen the muffins with a knife and serve.

Store any leftovers in an airtight container for up to 3 days, or freeze for up to a month.

Makes 1 dozen muffins.

Raspberry Muffins

Sweet, tart raspberries baked into vanilla-scented muffins make for an excellent rainy-day treat. Serve these for breakfast, at brunch, or for an afternoon tea—they'll make a delightfully sweet indulgence you'll return to again and again. For best results, use frozen, unsweetened raspberries (don't thaw); fresh are very delicate and will break down when you mix them into the batter. Serve these warm with some unsalted, grass-fed butter for a scrumptious, Paleo-style delight.

- 2 cups blanched almond flour
- 2 teaspoons baking soda
- 1/2 teaspoon sea salt
- 4 large eggs
- 1/2 cup coconut oil, melted
- 1/4 cup pure honey
- 1/2 cup unsweetened almond milk
- 1 cup frozen raspberries

Preheat oven to 350 degrees F.

In a large bowl, combine the almond flour, baking soda, and salt. Set aside.

In a mixing bowl, beat the eggs with the coconut oil, honey, and almond milk until light and smooth. Pour into the flour mixture, and stir until well combined. Fold in the frozen raspberries, being careful not to break them down too much.

Line a muffin tin with liners, and fill each cup 2/3 full of batter. Bake for 12–14 minutes, until tops are golden brown. Once cooled, loosen the muffins with a knife and serve.

Store any leftovers in an airtight container for up to 3 days. You can freeze these for weeks in a freezer bag for serving anytime.

Makes 1 dozen muffins.

Spiced Sweet Potato Muffins

These tender-crumbed muffins are full of flavor, thanks to rich spices like cinnamon, ginger, and clove. These muffins make an excellent choice for a fall brunch or even a holiday party, and can be served alongside a holiday meal in place of dinner rolls made with wheat flour. If you plan to serve them this way, reduce the maple syrup (for a more savory muffin), and they'll most definitely be the hit of the meal. For a more dessert-like finish, top these with some nuts of your choice.

- 2 cup blanched almond flour
- 1 teaspoon baking soda
- 1 teaspoon cinnamon
- 1/4 teaspoon ground nutmeg
- 1/4 teaspoon ground ginger
- 1/4 teaspoon ground cloves
- 1/2 teaspoon sea salt
- 2 large eggs
- 2 cups sweet potatoes, cooked and pureed
- 1/2 cup unsweetened almond milk
- 3 tablespoons pure maple syrup

Preheat oven to 350 degrees F.

In a large mixing bowl, combine the almond flour, baking soda, spices, and salt. Stir to combine.

In a small bowl, combine the eggs, pureed sweet potato, almond milk, and maple syrup. Beat until well combined. Add the wet ingredients to the flour mixture and mix well.

Line a muffin tin with liners, and fill each cup 2/3 full of batter. Bake for 12–14 minutes, until tops are golden brown. Once cooled, loosen the muffins with a knife and serve.

Store any leftovers in an airtight container or loosely wrapped in plastic for up to 3 days.

Makes 1 dozen muffins.

Mango Muffins

Mangos are the most widely eaten fruit in the world, and they taste delicious in these muffins—but they need to be sufficiently ripe. The easiest way to tell if it's ready is to smell the stem end. If it smells sweet and fruity, it is ready to be peeled and pitted. If it has no aroma, it needs another day or two to ripen up.

- 2 cups blanched almond flour
- 2 teaspoons baking soda
- 1/2 teaspoon sea salt
- 2 large eggs
- 1/2 cup coconut oil, melted
- 1/4 cup pure honey
- 1/2 cup unsweetened almond milk
- 1 ripe mango, pitted, peeled, and finely chopped
- 1/4 cup unsweetened coconut, shredded

Preheat oven to 350 degrees F.

In a large bowl, combine the almond flour, baking soda, and salt. Set aside.

In a mixing bowl, beat the eggs with the coconut oil, honey, and almond milk until light and smooth. Pour into the flour mixture, and stir until well combined. Fold in the finely chopped mango.

Line a muffin tin with liners, and fill each cup 2/3 full of batter. Sprinkle the coconut on top of the muffins.

Bake for 12–14 minutes, until tops are golden brown and coconut is lightly toasted. Once cooled, loosen the muffins with a knife and serve.

Store any leftovers in an airtight container for up to 3 days. You can freeze these for weeks in a freezer bag for serving anytime.

Makes 1 dozen muffins.

Cranberry Orange Muffins

These classic coffee shop muffins have been no friend of the Paleo diet—until now. These lightly sweet muffins are bursting with tart cranberries and are full of bright orange flavor. They're a great addition to a brunch display and perfect for a midday snack. Dried cherries make an appetizing substitute for the cranberries if you're looking for a variation. These muffins freeze beautifully, so it doesn't hurt to make a double batch and save some for later. Warm a muffin up in the microwave, slather it with some unsalted, grass-fed butter, and you'll be in fruit-filled heaven.

- 2 cups blanched almond flour
- 2 teaspoons baking soda
- 1/2 teaspoon sea salt
- 2 tablespoons orange zest
- 2 large eggs
- 1/2 cup unsalted, grass-fed butter, melted and cooled
- 1/4 cup pure honey
- 1/2 cup unsweetened almond milk
- 1/2 cup dried cranberries

Preheat oven to 350 degrees F.

In a large bowl, combine the almond flour, baking soda, salt, and orange zest. Set aside.

In a mixing bowl, beat the eggs with the butter, honey, and almond milk until light and smooth. Pour into the flour mixture, and stir until well combined. Fold in the dried cranberries.

Line a muffin tin with liners, and fill each cup 2/3 full of batter. Bake for 12–14 minutes, until tops are golden brown. Once cooled, loosen the muffins with a knife and serve.

Store any leftovers in an airtight container for up to 3 days. You can freeze these for weeks in a freezer bag for serving anytime.

Makes 1 dozen muffins.

Cherry Almond Muffins

Dark, sweet cherries are the star of these delightful muffins, and if you can find them in the frozen section of your supermarket, they're perfect for these honey-sweetened muffins topped with slivered almonds. If you can't find frozen, use fresh ones if you don't mind removing the pits. Dried cherries will work in a pinch, but they are no match for the flavor of fresh cherries. Freeze any leftovers for a delicious treat you can enjoy whenever the mood strikes.

- 2 cups blanched almond flour
- 2 teaspoons baking soda
- 1/2 teaspoon sea salt
- 4 large eggs
- 1/2 cup coconut oil, melted
- 1/4 cup pure honey
- 1/2 cup unsweetened almond milk
- 1 cup dark, sweet cherries, preferably frozen
- 1/2 cup almonds, sliced

Preheat oven to 350 degrees F.

In a large bowl, combine the almond flour, baking soda, and salt. Set aside.

In a mixing bowl, beat the eggs with the coconut oil, honey, and almond milk until light and smooth. Pour into the flour mixture, and stir until well combined. Fold in the cherries, being careful not to break them up.

Line a muffin tin with liners, and fill each cup 2/3 full of batter. Sprinkle the almonds over the top of the muffins. Bake for 12–14 minutes, until tops are golden brown. Once cooled, loosen the muffins with a knife and serve.

Store any leftovers in an airtight container for up to 3 days. You can freeze these for weeks in a freezer bag for serving anytime.

Makes 1 dozen muffins.

3

DESSERT MUFFINS

Paleo Almond Muffins

Lightly sweetened muffins topped with crunchy, slivered almonds make an excellent, sweet treat after a meal. These moist muffins are delicious with a bit of Paleo-approved jam, but they have plenty of flavor when eaten plain as well. One bite and you won't miss those sugary, high-carb bakery muffins anymore. You can easily freeze these, making a simple, grab-and-go Paleo snack.

- 2 cups blanched almond flour
- 2 teaspoons baking soda
- 1/2 teaspoon sea salt
- 4 large eggs
- 1/2 cup coconut oil, melted
- 1/4 cup pure honey
- 1 teaspoon almond extract
- 1/2 cup water
- 1/2 cup almond slices, toasted

Preheat oven to 350 degrees F.

Combine the almond flour, baking soda, and salt in a large bowl and set aside.

Beat the eggs with the coconut oil and honey, then add the almond extract and water, and stir to combine.

Line a muffin tin with liners, and fill each cup 2/3 full of batter, then sprinkle the almond slices on top. Bake for 10–12 minutes, until the muffins are lightly browned and the almonds lightly toasted.

Cool completely on a wire rack before removing the muffins from the pan. Serve with butter or Paleo-approved jam. Store leftover muffins in an airtight container or wrapped in plastic for up to 3 days.

Makes 1 dozen muffins.

Lemon Poppy Seed Muffins

These elegant muffins are fragrant with the scent of lemon, and thanks to the poppy seeds, boast a delicate bite. A step up from your traditional blueberry or banana, these simple-to-prepare muffins make an excellent brunch option, and also a terrific sweet treat after a meal when you don't want something too indulgent. For variety, orange zest works very well here, and you can even make them into mini muffins by using a mini muffin tin and baking for about half the time. Fill a basket, and they make a great gluten-free, Paleo-friendly gift. One bite of these beauties, and you'll never miss bakery muffins again!

- 2 cups blanched almond flour
- 2 teaspoons baking soda
- 1/2 teaspoon sea salt
- 3 large eggs
- 1/2 cup coconut oil, melted
- 1/4 cup pure honey
- Zest of 1 lemon
- 1/2 cup unsweetened almond milk
- 2 tablespoons poppy seeds

Preheat oven to 350 degrees F.

Combine the almond flour, baking soda, and salt in a large bowl and set aside.

Beat the eggs with the coconut oil and honey, then add the lemon zest and almond milk, and stir to combine. Fold in the poppy seeds.

Line a muffin tin with liners, and fill each cup 2/3 full of batter. Bake for 12–14 minutes, until tops are golden brown. Once cooled, loosen the muffins with a knife and serve.

Store any leftovers in an airtight container for up to 3 days.

Makes 1 dozen muffins.

Paleo Honey Muffins

Buttery, sweet, and tender, these delicious muffins are a cinch to prepare. While the recipe may seem plain, you'll be pleasantly surprised at the distinctive honey flavor. Serve them with unsalted, grass-fed butter and jam for a real treat, particularly for a Sunday brunch. For a twist, use a lightly fragrant varietal of honey—lavender or orange blossom, for example, work very nicely here. Whatever honey you use, be sure it is high quality, and you'll get a much nicer flavor.

- 2 cups blanched almond flour
- 2 teaspoons baking soda
- 1/2 teaspoon sea salt
- 4 large eggs
- 1/2 cup unsalted, grass-fed butter, melted and cooled
- 1/4 cup pure honey
- 1/2 cup unsweetened almond milk

Preheat oven to 350 degrees F.

In a large bowl, combine the almond flour, baking soda, and salt. Set aside.

In a mixing bowl, beat the eggs with the butter, honey, and almond milk until light and smooth. Pour into the flour mixture, and stir until well combined.

Line a muffin tin with liners, and fill each cup 2/3 full of batter. Bake for 12–14 minutes, until tops are golden brown. Once cooled, loosen the muffins with a knife and serve.

Store any leftovers in an airtight container for up to 3 days. You can freeze these for weeks in a freezer bag for serving anytime.

Makes 1 dozen muffins.

Simple Chocolate Muffins

*These easy-to-prepare chocolate muffins will surely satisfy your craving for
something chocolaty, while still keeping your Paleo diet on track. These
make an excellent dessert and will please even the most dire chocoholics. Use
natural cocoa powder instead of Dutch processed, as the method of processing
used violates the Paleo principles you've been working so hard to uphold. Buy
the highest-quality cocoa you can find for best results.*

- 2 cups blanched almond flour
- 1/2 cup unsweetened cocoa powder
- 1 teaspoon baking soda
- 1 teaspoon sea salt
- 2 large eggs
- 1/2 cup cold water
- 1 teaspoon pure vanilla extract
- 1/4 cup pure honey
- 1 cup walnuts, chopped (optional)

Preheat oven to 350 degrees F.

Mix together the almond flour, cocoa, baking soda, and salt in a bowl, and sift to combine well.

In a large bowl, beat the eggs until they are frothy. Add the water, vanilla, and honey, and beat until well combined.

Carefully pour the flour mixture into the wet ingredients, and stir until just combined. If using, fold half of the chopped walnuts into the batter.

Line a mini muffin tin with liners, or grease lightly with coconut oil, and fill each cup 2/3 full of batter. Sprinkle with the remaining walnuts, if using, and bake for 13–14 minutes. Muffins are done when the tops are firm and a toothpick inserted in the center of 1 comes out clean.

Cool before removing muffins from tin. Store any remaining muffins in an airtight container for up to 3 days.

Makes 1 dozen muffins.

Maple Pecan Muffins

Sweetened with real maple syrup, these are a welcome treat for late at night when you are hankering for something sweet but still want to stick to your diet. If you like, walnuts make a nice substitute for the pecans, although almost any type of nut will do. When buying maple syrup, make sure the product you select is real, pure maple syrup and not "pancake" syrup, which is just a fancy way of saying "high-fructose corn syrup with maple flavoring." Not only does it not taste as good, it is as far from Paleo-approved eating as it gets.

- 2 cups blanched almond flour
- 2 teaspoons baking soda
- 1/2 teaspoon sea salt
- 4 large eggs
- 1/2 cup unsalted, grass-fed butter, melted and cooled
- 1/4 cup pure maple syrup
- 1/2 cup unsweetened almond milk
- 1/2 cup raw pecans, chopped

Preheat oven to 350 degrees F.

In a large bowl, combine the almond flour, baking soda, and salt. Set aside.

In a mixing bowl, beat the eggs with the butter, maple syrup, and almond milk until light and smooth. Pour into the flour mixture, and stir until well combined.

Line a muffin tin with liners, and fill each cup 2/3 full of batter. Top each muffin with a few of the raw pecans. Bake for 12–14 minutes, until tops are golden brown and nuts are lightly toasted and fragrant. Once cooled, loosen the muffins with a knife and serve.

Store any leftovers in an airtight container for up to 3 days. You can freeze these for weeks in a freezer bag for serving anytime.

Makes 1 dozen muffins.

Chocolate Almond Butter Muffins

While peanut butter isn't a Paleo-approved diet food (peanuts are a legume, which is strictly prohibited on the plan), almond butter makes an excellent substitute. In this recipe, moist and tender chocolate muffins are filled with a dollop of almond butter. The result is similar to your favorite peanut butter cup, but it's Paleo approved. You'll absolutely love these chocolaty muffins with a hint of saltiness at their center. These are best served warm, so if you save leftovers, be sure to reheat them so the almond butter becomes soft and slightly melted.

- 2 cups blanched almond flour
- 1/2 cup unsweetened cocoa powder
- 1 teaspoon baking soda
- 1 teaspoon sea salt
- 2 large eggs
- 1/2 cup cold water
- 1 teaspoon pure vanilla extract
- 1/4 cup pure honey
- 12 teaspoons natural almond butter

Preheat oven to 350 degrees F.

Mix together the almond flour, cocoa, baking soda, and salt in a bowl, and sift to combine well.

In a large bowl, beat the eggs until they are frothy. Add the water, vanilla, and honey, and beat until well combined.

Carefully pour the flour mixture into the wet ingredients, and stir until just combined.

Line a mini muffin tin with liners, or grease lightly with coconut oil, and fill each cup 2/3 full of batter. Drop a teaspoon of almond butter in the center of each muffin.

Bake for 13–14 minutes. Muffins are done when the tops are firm and a toothpick inserted in the center of 1 comes out clean.

Allow the muffins to cool slightly before serving warm.

Store any remaining muffins in an airtight container for up to 3 days.

Makes 1 dozen muffins.

Vanilla Almond Muffins

Like your favorite biscotti, these deliciously fragrant muffins are best served with a cup of coffee or tea after a rich meal. Not particularly sweet, you'll be surprised at how successfully the light, vanilla flavor cures your craving for something sugary. While you can very often substitute other nuts in many muffin recipes, the delicate, slivered almonds in this one do an excellent job of complementing the subtle flavor of these muffins—other common nuts, such as walnuts or pecans, may overwhelm these.

- 2 cups blanched almond flour
- 2 teaspoons baking soda
- 1/2 teaspoon sea salt
- 4 large eggs
- 1/2 cup unsalted, grass-fed butter, melted and cooled
- 2 tablespoons pure honey
- 1/2 cup unsweetened almond milk
- 1 tablespoon pure vanilla extract
- 1 teaspoon pure almond extract
- 1/2 cup almonds, sliced

Preheat oven to 350 degrees F.

In a large bowl, combine the almond flour, baking soda, and salt. Set aside.

In a mixing bowl, beat the eggs with the butter, honey, almond milk, vanilla, and almond extract until light and smooth. Pour into the flour mixture, and stir until well combined.

Line a muffin tin with liners, and fill each cup 2/3 full of batter. Sprinkle the sliced almonds on top of the muffins. Bake for 12–14 minutes, until tops are golden brown and almonds are lightly toasted. Once cooled, loosen the muffins with a knife and serve.

Store any leftovers in an airtight container for up to 3 days. You can freeze these for weeks in a freezer bag for serving anytime.

Makes 1 dozen muffins.

Chocolate Coconut Muffins

These muffins are rich and moist, more like a fudge brownie than a muffin. The addition of shredded coconut pairs very well with the muffin's chocolate flavor, leaving you with a tender muffin that will rival even the best desserts. These are delicious at room temperature but even more indulgent when warm, so if yours have already cooled, a quick zap in the microwave will bring that warm, delicious flavor back.

- 1/2 cup coconut oil, melted
- 4 large eggs
- 2 teaspoons pure vanilla extract
- 2 tablespoons pure honey
- 1/2 cup blanched almond flour
- 1/4 cup unsweetened cocoa powder
- 1/2 cup unsweetened coconut, shredded, plus 2 tablespoons for topping
- 1 teaspoon baking soda

Preheat oven to 325 degrees F.

Beat the coconut oil with the eggs until you have a light yellow, frothy mixture. Add in the vanilla and honey.

In a large bowl, combine the almond flour, cocoa, 1/2 cup coconut, and baking soda. Add this to the egg mixture, and beat on low until just combined.

Line a muffin tin with liners, and fill each cup 2/3 full of batter. Top with the remaining coconut. Bake for 12–14 minutes, until tops are firm and a toothpick inserted in the center of 1 comes out clean. Once cooled, loosen the muffins with a knife and serve.

Store any leftovers in an airtight container for up to 3 days.

Makes 1 dozen muffins.

Blueberry Chocolate Chip Mini Muffins

Sometimes all it takes to satisfy your sweet tooth is one bite, and these bite-sized muffins, filled with juicy blueberries and rich, dark chocolate, will do the trick. While other berries and fruits are often paired with chocolate, blueberries with chocolate is often overlooked. The combination is not too sweet but not quite tart, and you'll love them. If you can find wild blueberries, they work especially well in mini muffins, ensuring a burst of fruit in every bite.

- 2 1/2 cups blanched almond flour
- 1 tablespoon coconut flour
- 1 teaspoon baking soda
- 1 teaspoon sea salt
- 1 stick unsalted, grass-fed butter, softened
- 1/2 cup pure honey
- 2 large eggs
- 1/2 cup unsweetened almond milk
- 1 tablespoon pure vanilla extract
- 1/2 cup fresh or frozen wild blueberries.
- 2 ounces dark chocolate or chocolate chips, finely chopped

Preheat oven to 350 degrees F.

Combine the almond flour, coconut flour, baking soda, and salt in a large bowl. Stir and set aside.

In a mixing bowl, beat the butter with the honey, and add the eggs, beating separately with each egg. On low speed add the almond milk and vanilla.

Add the flour mixture, and beat on low until just combined. Carefully fold in the blueberries and chocolate. Stir gently until well combined.

Line a mini muffin tin with liners, or grease lightly with coconut oil, and fill each cup 2/3 full of batter. Bake for 7–8 minutes, until tops are golden brown. Once cooled, loosen the muffins with a knife and serve.

Store any leftovers in an airtight container for up to 3 days.

Makes 2 dozen bite-sized muffins.

Double-Chocolate Cherry Muffins

Muffins can be more than breakfast, as you'll see with one bite of these lovelies. These intensely flavored muffins are a chocolate lover's delight. Moist and tender, these muffins are filled with high-quality chopped chocolate and dried cherries for a flavor combination you are sure to adore. For an extra element of richness, try adding chopped almonds or walnuts. Serve these dessert-like muffins after a meal for a delicious treat you or your guests will undoubtedly enjoy.

- 2 cups blanched almond flour
- 1/2 cup unsweetened cocoa powder
- 1 teaspoon sea salt
- 1 teaspoon baking soda
- 2 large eggs
- 1/2 cup cold water
- 1 teaspoon pure vanilla extract
- 1/4 cup pure honey
- 1/2 cup high-quality dark chocolate, chopped, or chocolate chips
- 1/2 cup dried cherries

Preheat oven to 350 degrees F.

Mix together the almond flour, cocoa, salt, and baking soda in a bowl, and sift to combine well.

In a large bowl, beat the eggs until they are frothy. Add the water, vanilla, and honey, and beat until well combined.

Carefully pour the flour mixture into the wet ingredients, and stir until just combined. Fold in the chopped chocolate and dried cherries.

Line a mini muffin tin with liners, or grease lightly with coconut oil, and fill each cup 2/3 full of batter. Bake for 13–14 minutes. Muffins are done when the tops are firm and a toothpick inserted in the center of 1 comes out clean.

Cool before removing muffins from tin. Store any remaining muffins in an airtight container for up to 3 days.

Makes 1 dozen muffins.

Double-Chocolate Peppermint Muffins

These rich, chocolate muffins with a hint of peppermint flavor are a huge hit at holiday parties or for a wintertime brunch you want to keep healthful. High-quality chocolate makes all the difference here, so don't skimp if you want the best flavor. While these are most tempting served warm, they can definitely be enjoyed at room temperature. Freeze any leftovers for a holiday treat any time of the year.

- 2 cups blanched almond flour
- 1/2 cup unsweetened cocoa powder
- 1 teaspoon baking soda
- 1 teaspoon sea salt
- 2 large eggs
- 1/2 cup cold water
- 2 teaspoons pure peppermint extract
- 1/4 cup pure honey
- 1/2 cup high-quality dark chocolate, chopped, or chocolate chips

Preheat oven to 350 degrees F.

Mix together the almond flour, cocoa, baking soda, and salt in a bowl, and sift to combine well.

In a large bowl, beat the eggs until they are frothy. Add the water, peppermint extract, and honey, and beat until well combined.

Carefully pour the flour mixture into the wet ingredients, and stir until just combined. Fold in the chopped chocolate.

Line a mini muffin tin with liners, or grease lightly with coconut oil, and fill each cup 2/3 full of batter. Bake for 13–14 minutes. Muffins are done when the tops are firm and a toothpick inserted in the center of 1 comes out clean.

Cool before removing muffins from tin. Store any remaining muffins in an airtight container for up to 3 days.

Makes 1 dozen muffins.

Key Lime Coconut Muffins

Sometimes you want a dessert, but not necessarily something rich and filled with chocolate. These key lime delights provide a light-and-easy, dessert-like experience that will have you dreaming of your next beach getaway. If you can't find key limes (they're particularly small and usually sold in bags), regular limes will do, but you'll be amazed at the difference in flavor between the two.

- 2 cups blanched almond flour
- 2 teaspoons baking soda
- 1/2 teaspoon sea salt
- 2 teaspoons key lime zest
- 2 large eggs
- 1/2 cup coconut oil, melted
- 1/4 cup pure honey
- 1/2 cup coconut milk
- 2 tablespoons key lime juice
- 1/4 cup unsweetened coconut, shredded

Preheat oven to 350 degrees F.

In a large bowl, combine the almond flour, baking soda, salt, and lime zest. Set aside.

In a mixing bowl, beat the eggs with the coconut oil, honey, coconut milk, and lime juice until light and smooth. Pour into the flour mixture, and stir until well combined.

Line a muffin tin with liners, and fill each cup 2/3 full of batter. Top each with a sprinkle of shredded coconut. Bake for 12–14 minutes, until tops are golden brown. Once cooled, loosen the muffins with a knife and serve.

Store any leftovers in an airtight container for up to 3 days. You can freeze these for weeks in a freezer bag for serving anytime.

Makes 1 dozen muffins.

Browned-Butter Honey Muffins

These honey-sweetened muffins get their amazing depth of flavor from unsalted, grass-fed butter browned in a skillet. When butter is handled this way, it takes on a nuttiness that is hard to match elsewhere. While you can add nuts or spices to this recipe with much success, try the muffins first as they are; you may be surprised at just how delicious these seemingly plain muffins can be. Use a stainless steel or other light-colored skillet when you brown the butter—it can be difficult to tell when it reaches the right color in a dark pan.

- 1/2 cup unsalted, grass-fed butter
- 2 cups blanched almond flour
- 2 teaspoons baking soda
- 1/2 teaspoon sea salt
- 4 large eggs
- 1/4 cup pure honey
- 1/2 cup unsweetened almond milk

Preheat oven to 350 degrees F.

In a medium skillet, heat the butter over medium-low heat. Cook it until it is dark brown and foamy, with brown bits on the bottom. It will be nice and fragrant as well. Once it is brown, immediately pour it into a bowl or measuring cup to cool. Allow to cool for about 10 minutes.

In a large bowl, combine the almond flour, baking soda, and salt. Set aside.

In a mixing bowl, beat the eggs with the browned butter, honey, and almond milk until light and smooth. Pour into the flour mixture, and stir until well combined.

Line a muffin tin with liners, and fill each cup 2/3 full of batter. Bake for 12–14 minutes, until tops are golden brown. Once cooled, loosen the muffins with a knife and serve.

Store any leftovers in an airtight container for up to 3 days. You can freeze these for weeks in a freezer bag for serving anytime.

Makes 1 dozen muffins.

Chocolate Chip Banana Muffins

The combination of chocolate and banana is a favorite for adults and kids alike, and this easy recipe incorporates both flavors well, while adhering to the Paleo diet. These make a perfect, Paleo-friendly treat when you want something sweet, and a nice dessert when you'd like a little taste of chocolate after a meal. Freeze leftovers for a chocolaty snack anytime you feel the urge.

- 2 1/2 cups blanched almond flour
- 1 teaspoon baking soda
- 1/2 teaspoon sea salt
- 2 large eggs
- 2 medium, ripe bananas, mashed
- 1/2 cup water
- 2 teaspoons pure vanilla extract
- 1/4 cup pure honey
- 1/2 cup high-quality dark chocolate, chopped, or chocolate chips

Preheat oven to 350 degrees F.

Mix together the almond flour, baking soda, and salt in a bowl, and sift to combine well.

In a large bowl, beat the eggs with the bananas. Add the water, vanilla extract, and honey, and beat until well combined.

Carefully pour the flour mixture into the wet ingredients, and stir until just combined. Fold in the chopped chocolate.

Fill greased or lined muffin tins 2/3 full, and bake for 13–14 minutes. Muffins are done when the tops are firm and a toothpick inserted in the center of 1 comes out clean.

Cool before removing muffins from tin. Store any remaining muffins in an airtight container for up to 3 days.

Makes 1 dozen muffins.

The Basics of the Paleo Diet

- **Chapter 4**: What Is the Paleo Diet?

- **Chapter 5**: The Benefits of Paleo

- **Chapter 6**: The Trouble with Gluten

- **Chapter 7**: Paleo Food Guide

4

WHAT IS THE PALEO DIET?

Whether modern healthcare professionals want to admit it or not, the Paleo diet closely mirrors what most of them tell their patients: eat more fruits, vegetables, and lean meats, and stay away from processed garbage. The diet, also known as the Stone Age diet, the caveman diet, and the hunter-gatherer diet, has gained a significant following in recent years, and there's some pretty good research to support the switch.

How Did the Paleo Diet Start?

Back in the 1970s a gastroenterologist by the name of Walter L. Voegtlin observed that digestive diseases such as colitis, Crohn's disease, and irritable bowel syndrome were much more prevalent in people who followed a modern Western diet than it was in people's ancestors, whose diet consisted largely of vegetables, fruits, nuts, and lean meats. He began treating patients with these disorders by recommending diets low in carbohydrates and high in animal fats.

Unfortunately, the medical world simply wasn't ready to give up the idea that a low-fat, low-calorie diet was the healthiest way to eat, so

Dr. Voegtlin's observations and research went largely unnoticed, and the Paleo diet was shoved to the back of the drawer.

Finally—The Stone Age Is Cool Again!

Fast forward a decade to a point when medical researchers had gained considerably more insight into how the human body actually works. Melvin Konner, S. Boyd Eaton, and Marjorie Shostak of Emory University published a book called *The Paleolithic Prescription: A Program of Diet and Exercise and a Design for Living*, then followed it up with a second book, *The Stone-Age Health Programme: Diet and Exercise as Nature Intended*. The first book became the foundation for most of the modern versions of the Paleo diet, and the second backed it up with more research.

The main difference was that instead of eliminating any foods that people's ancestors wouldn't have had access to as Dr. Voegtlin did originally, Konner, Eaton, and Shostak encouraged eating foods that were nutritionally and proportionally similar to a traditional caveman diet. Because it was more realistic, the diet caught on like wildfire, and the research in favor of it continues to grow.

What Are the Rules?

Paleo is one of the easiest diets on the planet to follow: just remember to keep it real. If it's processed, artificial, or otherwise not directly from the earth, don't eat it. It's that simple. Here's a list of the delicious, healthful foods that the Paleo diet encourages:

- Eggs
- Healthful oils—olive and coconut are best; canola oil is under debate right now, too
- Lean animal proteins
- Nuts and seeds (note, however, that peanuts are NOT nuts)

- Organic fruits
- Organic vegetables
- Seafood, especially cold-water fish such as salmon and tuna in order to get the most omega-3 fatty acids

Sounds kind of familiar, doesn't it? That's because it's probably what your doctor encouraged you to eat more of the last time that you went to see him or her! Now let's take a look at some foods that are off the table if you're going to eat Stone Age style:

- Alcohol
- Artificial foods, such as preservatives and zero-calorie sweeteners
- Cereal grains, such as wheat, barley, hops, corn, oats, rye, and rice
- Dairy (though some followers allow dairy for the health benefits)
- Legumes (including peanuts)
- Processed foods, such as wheat flour and sugar
- Processed meats, such as bacon, deli meats, sausage, and canned meats
- Starchy vegetables (though these are currently under debate)

Frequently Asked Questions

Now that you have a general idea of what you can and can't eat, you may still have a few questions, so here's a list of those most frequently asked.

Q. Why do I have to quit drinking?

A. Beer is basically liquid grain, and it's packed with empty calories. Many types of alcoholic products contain gluten, which is discussed in detail in Chapter 6. Mixed drinks and wine are often loaded with sugar. If you absolutely can't go without that Friday-night cocktail, shoot for red wine, tequila, potato vodka, or white rum—and be careful what you mix it with.

Q. Why are legumes forbidden? They're natural foods and great sources of protein.

A. Most legumes, in their raw state, are toxic. They contain lectins—proteins that bind carbohydrates and have been shown to cause such autoimmune diseases as lupus and rheumatoid arthritis. The phytates in many legumes inhibit your absorption of critical minerals, and the protease inhibitors interfere with how your body breaks down protein.

Q. Why no dairy?

A. This one's under debate and there are many Paleo followers who still incorporate dairy regularly into their diets. The main reason that dairy is generally forbidden is that humans are the only animals who drink milk as adults, and many food allergies and digestive disorders are lactose related. There's a much more scientific answer for this question, but it boils down to believing or not believing that milk is bad for you.

Q. How will I lose weight eating fat?

A. This is a question that most people have initially because you're programmed to believe that red meat is bad for your heart. The fact is lean, organic, free-range meat is an excellent source of protein and many other vitamins and minerals. You're not going to be living on it alone; you're going to be incorporating it into a healthful diet.

Q. Peanuts are nuts and corn is a vegetable, so why are they off-limits?

A. *Au contraire.* Peanuts are legumes and corn is a grain. Be careful that you know what food groups everything you eat falls into or you may sabotage your efforts to be healthier.

THE BENEFITS OF PALEO

Many people turn to the Paleo diet because of the weight-loss benefits, but that's not where the idea originated. If you remember, the diet was created by a gastroenterologist to help his patients with various gastric disorders. Of course, weight loss is a wonderful side effect that has its own set of healthful benefits.

When you add in the myriad other perks, going caveman is almost a no-brainer. Let's take a quick peek at some of the biggest health benefits of following a Paleo diet.

Weight Loss

Since this is one of the primary reasons that many people decide to switch to a Paleo diet, this is a good place to start. Because you're eliminating empty carbs and adding in lots of healthful plant fiber and lean protein, losing weight will be much easier. A few other factors that contribute to healthful weight loss include:

- Plant fiber takes longer to digest, so you feel full longer.
- Lean proteins help keep your energy levels steady while you build muscle.

- Omega-3s help boost your metabolism and reduce body fat.
- You'll be eating a greater volume of food but taking in fewer calories.

The bottom line is that you'll be consuming foods that help your body function the way that it's supposed to, and one of the natural side effects of that is weight loss.

Healthy Digestive System

Remember that this was the original reason for the diet to be utilized. The theory is that people's bodies aren't adapted to eating grains, dairy, and other foods that are forbidden by the Paleo diet, and so they cause digestive upset, inflammation, and discomfort. Also, your digestive tract needs fiber to help it sweep food through your system or else it builds up and causes problems. Just some of the conditions that may be improved by going caveman include:

- Colitis
- Constipation
- Gas
- Heartburn
- Irritable bowel syndrome

Many people who begin the Paleo diet for other reasons, such as weight loss or heart health, report improved digestive health. Yet another reason that this incredible diet is worth your time!

Type 2 Diabetes Prevention

In the United States and other cultures that have adopted a Western diet, type 2 diabetes has reached disastrous proportions. Historically an adult disease, children are developing this debilitating illness at an alarming rate, and there's no sign of this trend changing. One of the main culprits is excess consumption of processed sugars and flours.

By simply eliminating these calorie-laden, nutritionless foods from your diet, you can literally save your own life. The Paleo diet helps you avoid type 2 diabetes as well as metabolic syndrome, a precursor to many different diseases, for the following reasons:

- Omega-3s help reduce belly fat, an indicator of diabetes and metabolic syndrome.
- Lean proteins and plant fiber help increase insulin resistance so that your sugar levels don't spike.
- The vitamin C that's so readily available in citrus fruits and colorful veggies helps reduce belly fat.
- Lean protein takes longer to metabolize so you avoid energy highs and lows.

Immune Health

When you eat foods that your body isn't adapted to, such as processed grains, legumes, and dairy products, your body produces an allergic response in the form of inflammation, even if you don't experience any obvious outward symptoms. You may notice dark circles under your eyes as well as a feeling of general lethargy. You may attribute these symptoms to stress or exhaustion, but they're actually signs of a chronic allergy.

Inflammation in your body is a bad thing if it's occurring chronically, and it has been causally linked to such autoimmune disorders as:

- Fibromyalgia
- Lupus
- Multiple sclerosis
- Rheumatoid arthritis
- Several different types of cancer

The sad part here is that you don't even realize what you're doing to your body because there are often no symptoms until you have developed the disease. Switching to the Paleo diet may help reduce or eliminate your risk of many debilitating illnesses.

Cardiovascular Health

For most of your life, you've probably been told how horrible red meat and other animal proteins are for your heart, but recent research indicates that this is simply not true. Remember that there's a huge difference in scarfing down a fatty hamburger or sausage and enjoying a lean, organic, grass-fed steak. The burger and sausage are full of saturated fats and, most likely, hormones and additives.

On the other hand, steak is a lean, nutritious protein that delivers essential vitamins and minerals with very little bad fat and no empty calories, preservatives, or hormones. When you throw omega-3s and LDL-lowering healthful fats into the mix, you've got a heart-healthful meal that's good for anybody.

A Few Final Words on Health

The health benefits of giving up processed flour, refined sugar, and foods that cause inflammatory responses could fill an entire doctoral thesis, and the advantages to eliminating hormones and artificial additives from foods could fill another one. This chapter didn't even touch on how a Paleo diet can help with allergies, cancer, brain health, joint health, or celiac disease, but some of these will be covered in the discussion of the health risks of gluten in the next chapter. Suffice to say, the benefits of going Paleo far outweigh the relatively minor inconvenience of giving up a few foods.

6

THE TROUBLE WITH GLUTEN

Of the many health benefits of switching to a Paleo diet, one of the main benefits is that foods allowed on the diet don't have gluten in them. For millions of people worldwide, eating caveman-style is a relatively simple way to avoid digestive upset and even cancers that are caused by an allergy to gluten.

What Is Gluten?

Latin for "glue," gluten is a protein found in wheat and grains that gives the ground flours elasticity and helps them to rise. It's also the binding component that gives bread its chewy texture and keeps it from crumbling apart after baking. Because gluten is insoluble in water, it can be removed from flour, but typically when you do that, you lose all of the good properties that make breads and cakes what they are.

Without gluten, your baked goods won't rise and they'll have a grainy, crumbly texture. They won't taste anything like their gluten-laden cousins, and you probably won't want to eat more after the first bite. Because of an increasing demand for gluten-free products, food corporations have dedicated a tremendous amount of time and money into creating tasty, effective gluten-free products. Unfortunately, most commercially prepared gluten-free recipe mixes still fall short.

Is the Paleo Diet Gluten-Free?

Because gluten naturally occurs in wheat and grains, the Paleo diet is completely gluten-free. All grain products are strictly forbidden. Remember, the original creator of the diet was a gastroenterologist developing a plan that would help his patients with gastric disorders. Gluten intolerance is one of the most prevalent causes of gastrointestinal distress in Western civilization.

What Is Gluten Intolerance?

Gluten intolerance, or celiac disease in its advanced stage, is a condition that damages the small intestine, and it's triggered by eating foods that have gluten in them. Some of these foods include:

- Bread
- Cookies
- Just about any baked goods
- Most flours, including white and wheat flours
- Pasta
- Pizza dough

Gluten triggers an immune response in the small intestine that causes damage to its inside. This can lead to an inability to absorb vital nutrients. Other illnesses associated with this disease include lactose intolerance, bone loss, several types of cancer, neurological complications, and malnutrition.

Diseases notwithstanding, just the symptoms of gluten intolerance can disrupt daily life. They include:

- Depression
- Fatigue
- Joint pain
- Neuropathy
- Osteoporosis
- Rashes
- Severe diarrhea
- Stomach cramps

These are only a few of the symptoms that a person with gluten intolerance can suffer from, and since all foods that contain gluten are forbidden on the Paleo diet, you can see what the appeal is.

The Harmful Effects of Gluten

Gluten doesn't just harm people with fully developed celiac disease. It's actually harmful to us all. Long-term studies indicate that people who have even a mild sensitivity to gluten exhibit a significantly higher risk of death than people who do not. The worst part is that 99 percent of people with gluten sensitivity don't even know they have it. They attribute their symptoms to other conditions, such as stress or fatigue.

Absorption Malfunction

One of the attributes that many obese or overweight people share is the fact that they can still feel hungry after eating a full meal. This feeling of hunger is because gluten sensitivity is preventing your body from absorbing vital nutrients.

Food Addiction

There are chemicals called exorphins in some foods that cause you to crave food even when you're not hungry. Food addiction is a serious issue and doesn't necessarily denote a lack of willpower; these exorphins are actually a drug-like chemical released in your brain that creates an irresistible desire for more food. Gluten contains as many as fifteen different exorphins.

Though food companies have created gluten-free foods, they often replace the gluten with flavor-enhancers, such as sodium and sugar, which can still seriously sabotage your dieting and fitness efforts. Another advantage to the Paleo diet is that by following it, you're not only eliminating gluten, you're also avoiding the pitfalls of commercially prepared foods that continue to make you sick.

Other Conditions Related to Gluten

There are numerous other conditions related to gluten sensitivity, and many professionals postulate that this is simply because people's bodies aren't adapted to eating grains so they are treated as allergens. Other symptoms or disorders linked to eating gluten include:

- Anxiety
- Autism
- Dementia
- Migraines
- Mouth sores
- Schizophrenia
- Seizures

These aren't just minor aches and pains, though gluten sensitivity can cause those, too. These are major diseases and conditions that can ruin your life. It's no wonder that people who know that they suffer from gluten intolerance consider the Paleo diet.

Health Benefits of Going Gluten-Free

Obviously, there are countless benefits of giving up gluten, but here are a few that may be of particular interest to you:

- Decreased chance of several types of cancer
- Healthy, painless digestion
- Healthy skin
- Improved brain function
- Improved mood
- Reduced appetite
- Weight loss (or gain, if you're underweight because of malnutrition)

With the obvious advantages of giving up grains, it's difficult to understand exactly why people would hesitate. It's just a matter of making some adjustments to your diet, and now that understanding about both food and health is increasing, there are some great alternatives out there that will help you get rid of your addiction to grains!

PALEO FOOD GUIDE

S hopping for foods that are Paleo friendly can be a daunting task
when you're first starting out. What's allowed and what's not? What
are all of those mystery ingredients that are listed in foods? For the
most part, stocking your fridge and pantry is fairly simple, but there
are going to be times when you don't want to eat just steak and broc-
coli, and there will be other times when you need something fast and
simple. Don't worry: you'll get the hang of it.

There are a few different versions of the Paleo diet, but this discussion will focus on the modern middle road so that it's easier for you
to make the transition to your new, healthier lifestyle. Throughout the
following paragraphs, you'll learn what foods are OK and where you
can find them. You'll also learn some alternate ingredients for baking
muffins and other goodies that won't get you kicked out of the cave!

Paleo Pantry and Kitchen Tips

The first bit of good news is that you're not going to be counting calories.
Instead, you're going to try to keep your portions in line with what your
ancestors most likely ate. A diet that consists of 50 to 60 percent protein,
30 to 45 percent healthful carbs, and 5 to 10 percent healthful vegetable
fats, such as olive oil, avocados, nuts, and seeds, is the general goal.

Basically, when you're stacking your plate, put your protein on one side and your fruits and veggies on the other. Snacks can be whatever you want, but veggies and nuts are great choices. Be careful with nuts and fruits; though they're good for you, they're high in calories and can sabotage your weight-loss efforts if you're not careful.

If Possible, Go Raw

Many fruits and vegetables lose nutritional value when you cook them, so when possible, eat them raw. You'll also eat less because you'll be chewing more. If you opt to cook your veggies, steam them lightly so they maintain their bright colors. A key clue that you've cooked your greens to death is that they've lost that pretty vibrant green hue and turned an olive color. Try to avoid that.

Steaming, baking, grilling, and broiling are all great methods of cooking and require little added fat to prevent sticking. It should go without saying that the fryer can be retired to the garage to be sold at your next rummage sale.

Cooking on the Fly

Meals away from home can be a real challenge when you're first starting out. Restaurants are filled with tempting burgers and fries, and you have no idea what's in the salad dressings. If you must eat out, order a plain garden salad with oil and vinegar. You could also request a steak or chicken breast to go on top, but make sure that they either grill it dry or use olive oil.

Opt not to eat out in the beginning. Instead, make an amazing soup at home for dinner with enough leftover that you aren't tempted to go out for a quick fix. That way, you know what's in your food and you know that it's going to be delicious!

Plan Ahead

If you know in advance what you're going to eat for lunch or for dinner, you're not going to be as likely to cheat with something quick from the vending machine. Take snacks to work with you so that the box of doughnuts isn't so tempting.

Meats and Proteins

Your meats need to come from grass-fed, organic livestock, free-range poultry, or wild-caught fish and seafood. Wild game is great, too, if you're so inclined. Actually, meats such as venison are extremely low in bad fats and high in good fats and lean protein, so feel free to partake!

Fruits and Vegetables

If at all possible, shop at your local farmers' market for fresh organic fruits and veggies. Since the Paleo diet is dependent upon your creativity to complete a hot, fresh, delicious meal without the aid of flours, fats, and no-no's, you're going to have to learn a number of ways to prepare dishes. Plus, if you're offering a wide variety of foods that your family knows and loves, you won't be under so much pressure to create a single main dish that everybody will eat and enjoy.

Tomatoes are a great addition to any salad and make a flavorful base for soups and sauces. They're packed with nutrients and have so many uses that you should always have some on hand. Other staples should include carrots, peppers, cauliflower, and celery.

For fruits, opt for ones that are high in nutrients and relatively low in sugar, such as stone fruits and berries. Berries are also fabulous sources of antioxidants, phytonutrients, and vitamins. Apples are an easy grab-and-go food, as are peaches, oranges, and bananas. The dark tip of the banana that you usually pick off is rich in vitamin K, so eat it!

Oils and Fats

Oils high in saturated fats, such as corn oil and vegetable oil, are out. Opt instead for oils that are high in omega-3s, such as olive oil, avocado oil, coconut oil, and possibly canola oil. The latter is currently a point of contention among long-term Paleo followers, but there's a compelling argument to include it.

Seasonings

Your success with making the transition to the caveman way of eating is largely dependent on how flavorful your food is. As a result, you're going to need to incorporate various herbs and spices to make your dishes delicious. Here are a few that you should always have on hand:

- Allspice
- Black pepper
- Basil
- Cayenne pepper
- Cinnamon
- Cloves
- Crushed red pepper
- Curry powder
- Dry mustard
- Garlic—fresh and powdered
- Mustard seed
- Oregano
- Paprika
- Parsley
- Rosemary
- Thyme

Snacks

Finally, you'll probably want to keep some snacks on hand. Now, that does NOT mean cupcakes, potato chips, or crackers. However, there are still many options, such as certain beef jerky (or even better, make your own!), dried fruits, nuts, and seeds. They're satisfying and add nutrients to your diet instead of unhealthful fats.

Paleo Shopping Tips

Going to the grocery store is going to be a bit of a challenge at first, just as it is anytime that you make changes to your diet. Especially if you're accustomed to eating a large amount of refined flour and sugar and aren't yet over your sugar addiction, it's not going to be easy. Here are a few tips to help you along your way.

- Shop for your produce at the local farmers' market if possible.
- When at the grocery store, shop around the perimeter of the store. That's where most stores keep all of their meats and produce, and 99 percent of your food is going to come from those departments. If you need to get something from an aisle, go straight in, get it, and get back to the perimeter before those cookies catch your eye!
- Make a list and stick to it.
- If you do choose to eat canned fruits and veggies, make sure that you read the label so that you're not getting hidden sodium and preservatives.
- Buy meat in bulk when you catch a sale.
- Don't shop hungry! Have a low-fat, high-protein snack before you go so that you aren't tempted while you're there.

CONCLUSION

M aking any kind of a dietary change can be challenging, especially when it involves giving up foods you love. Because the Paleo diet is still relatively new to the health and wellness community, it's often misunderstood and therefore discarded because of its seeming restrictiveness. However, those who understand the theory recognize that it's sound, and once you actually begin practicing it, you'll realize that the only real restrictions are ones you place upon yourself. You just need to be a little bit creative!

Because the Paleo diet was created by a gastroenterologist specifically to help his patients regain good health, you're going to experience some wonderful health benefits. Even if you made the switch only to lose weight, you're going to find that you feel better, have more energy, and perhaps even notice such benefits as clearer skin and improved digestion.

Now that you understand how to make muffins that are Paleo friendly, you have even more culinary options and can rest assured that eating healthfully doesn't always mean sacrificing foods you enjoy. These Paleo muffin recipes will provide a solid foundation for your baking adventures to come: use them as they are, or modify them to suit your particular tastes—if you like, they can simply serve as a guideline and springboard for your imagination

As you become more comfortable eating caveman style, you're going to start thinking of ways to incorporate all of the delicious fruits and vegetables into your diet in original, flavorful ways. You'll probably also start to consider how you can transform your old, fattening recipes into something Paleo-worthy.

Ready availability of ingredients such as almond flour, almond milk, honey, and blackstrap molasses make it easy for you to experiment with your own healthful ingredients. If you're a blueberry–chocolate chip type, toss some bittersweet chocolate pieces into your recipe along with those plump, disease-fighting blue orbs. If carrot cake is your thing, tweak your recipe using the methods you've learned in this book.

Regardless of whether you prefer nuts, fruits, vegetables, or any combination thereof, there's probably a healthful, Paleo-friendly muffin recipe out there just waiting for you to try it. If not, why not invent one and share it with others?

Hopefully you enjoy these muffin recipes, and may you eat them in the best of health!

RESOURCES

Alternative Ingredients for Baking Paleo

Almond milk: Widely available in your grocer's dairy case, almond milk is a healthful, delicious replacement for dairy, consisting simply of ground almonds and filtered water. Characterized by an extremely mild, nutty flavor, almond milk is high in protein and low in bad fats. Unless stated otherwise, most brands contain added sweeteners, so be sure to buy unsweetened varieties.

Blanched almond flour: This is perhaps one of the most important ingredients in Paleo baking. While there are some other flours that are usable, blanched almond flour, in which the skins have been removed and the almonds ground to a fine flour, is hard to beat, and lends a mildly nutty flavor to your recipes. You can also make your own in a powerful blender or food processor by grinding almonds to flour, although it's difficult to know when to stop to avoid creating almond butter. Almond flour is high in protein and fiber and contains many more nutrients than refined, grain-based flours. Note that almond flour is different from almond meal, which is coarser in texture, and will not give you the best results when baking. Usually available at most grocery stores in the baking section; otherwise, check Amazon.com.

Cocoa powder: Unsweetened, natural cocoa powder. Available in grocery stores nationwide, but for higher-quality brands, check your local natural foods store or Amazon.com.

Coconut flour: Made from dried coconut that is ground into flour, coconut flour is extremely high in fiber and low in digestible carbs. Due to its high-fiber content, it's great as a weight-loss aid. However, coconut flour is rarely used as the sole flour for baking and should not be substituted for almond flour unless specifically stated. May not be available at your local grocer; check your local natural foods store or Amazon.com.

Coconut milk: You'll want to use canned, full-fat coconut milk in cookie recipes, unless otherwise noted. Coconut milk in a carton is made for drinking and is lightened up with water. In addition to its rich, sweet flavor, coconut milk boasts numerous health benefits, including maintenance of stable blood sugar and promotion of cardiovascular, bone, muscle, and nerve health. Often found in the Asian section of your grocery store. Native Forest makes a BPA-free version.

Coconut oil: An excellent butter substitute with a light but distinct coconut flavor. When purchasing, be sure to buy unrefined, virgin coconut oil. Coconut oil boasts a wide range of health benefits—good for your heart, your digestion, and your immune system, it is also useful in helping with weight loss. Melt in the microwave before measuring, and beware that mixing it with cold ingredients may cause it to seize up. Can be purchased at most grocery stores.

Coconut, shredded and unsweetened: Most shredded coconut you'll find in the baking section of your grocery store is sweetened with refined sugars, so make sure the package says unsweetened. May need to be purchased at a health food store.

Coconut sugar: Also known as palm sugar, coconut sugar is a sweetener made from coconut. You can find it at your local health food store or Amazon.com.

Extracts: When using flavorings and extracts, such as vanilla, almond, or lemon, make sure to buy only pure, natural extracts. Artificial versions have chemicals and additives that do not adhere to the Paleo diet. Most are available at your local grocer.

Honey: Pure, raw honey is the best sweetener for the recipes in this book. Be careful of flavored varieties, as the scent may come out in the final product. Locally produced honey purchased at farmer's markets or a natural foods store is best.

Leavening agents: Baking soda, baking powder, and cream of tartar are common items, although baking powder may be avoided in Paleo recipes, as it contains cornstarch. All of these are available in the baking aisle of your local grocery store.

Maple syrup: Always buy pure maple syrup, and make sure it states this on the container. National brands or any brands marked "pancake syrup" are simply maple-flavored, high-fructose corn syrup and should be avoided.

Palm shortening: A natural, vegetable-based, non-hydrogenated shortening that does not contain the trans fats of traditional versions. Great for replacing butter, it makes excellent frosting. May be available at your local grocer; otherwise, check your local health food store.

Salt: When using salt for Paleo baking, it's important to use a good sea salt instead of traditional table salt, which contains additives and preservatives. Keep in mind that even if you generally avoid salt, a small amount may be required for some leavening agents to work properly.

Sources/Brands

Amazon is a Web marketplace where you can find products of all types. Most of the items you need for this book can be found at Amazon.com, and sometimes for lower prices than you'll find locally.

Bob's Red Mill is an all-natural brand of gluten-free flours, shredded coconut, and other dried or powdered ingredients. You can find many of their products in your local grocery store's baking aisle, or at BobsRedMill.com.

Celtic Sea Salt is a maker of authentic, unprocessed sea salt, which will enhance the flavors of your baked goods. Go to CelticSeaSalt.com for more information on their products as well as where to buy.

Coconut Secrets makes a wide variety of all-natural products out of coconut. You'll find coconut flour, coconut oil, and other heart-healthful coconut products at CoconutSecret.com.

Penzeys is a retailer of high-quality spices and flavorings, including high-quality extracts and cocoa powder. Go to Penzeys.com for more information.

Spectrum is a brand of all-natural, organic oils available at grocers nationwide. Go to SpectrumOrganics.com for more information on their coconut oil, palm shortening, and other high-quality products.

Tropical Traditions is a maker of high-quality coconut products, such as oil or flour. Go to TropicalTraditions.com for more information.

Whole Foods Market is the world's largest natural foods store, with a variety of gluten-free and Paleo-friendly products. For locations, go to WholeFoodsMarket.com.

Made in the USA
San Bernardino, CA
01 March 2014